Plant-Based Cooking Guide

50 Simple and Tasty Recipes to Improve your Health

Lily Mullen

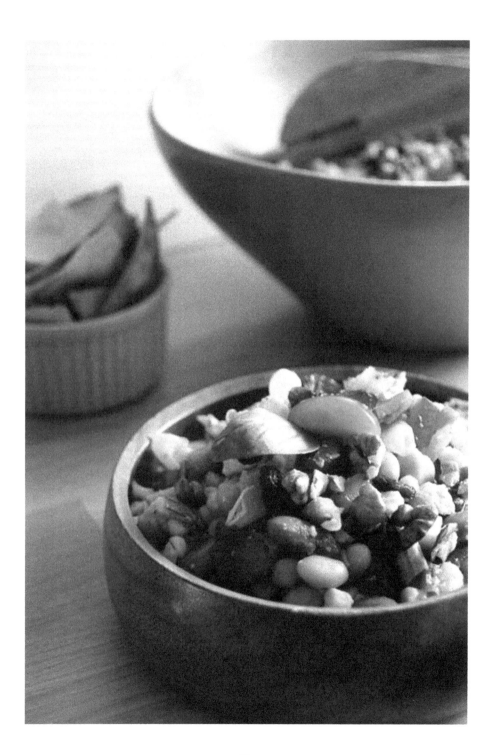

indirect, which are incurred as a result of the use of information contained within this document, including, but not limited to, — errors, omissions, or inaccuracies.

TABLE OF CONTENTS

Introduction

A plant-based eating routine backing and upgrades the entirety of this. For what reason should most of what we eat originate from the beginning?

Eating more plants is the first nourishing convention known to man to counteract and even turn around the ceaseless diseases that assault our general public.

Plants and vegetables are brimming with large scale and micronutrients that give our bodies all that we require for a sound and productive life. By eating, at any rate, two suppers stuffed with veggies consistently, and nibbling on foods grown from the ground in the middle of, the nature of your wellbeing and at last your life will improve.

The most widely recognized wellbeing worries that individuals have can be reduced by this one straightforward advance.

Things like weight, inadequate rest, awful skin, quickened maturing, irritation, physical torment, and absence of vitality would all be able to be decidedly influenced by expanding the admission of plants and characteristic nourishments.

If you're reading this book, then you're probably on a journey to get healthy because you know good health and nutrition go hand in hand.

Maybe you're looking at the plant-based diet as a solution to those love handles.

Whatever the case may be, the standard American diet millions of people eat daily is not the best way to fuel your body.

If you ask me, any other diet will already be a significant improvement. Since what you eat fuels your body, you can imagine that eating junk will make you feel just that—like junk.

I've followed the standard American diet for several years: my plate was loaded with high-fat and carbohydrate-rich foods. I know this doesn't sound like a horrible way to eat, but keep in mind that most Americans don't focus on eating healthy fats and complex carbs—we live on processed foods.

The consequences of eating foods filled with trans fats, preservatives, and mountains of sugar are fatigue, reduced mental focus, mood swings, and weight gain. To top it off, there's the issue of opening yourself up to certain diseases— some life-threatening—when you neglect paying attention to what you eat .

Vegan King Salad

Preparation time: 10 minutes

Cooking time: 30 minutes

Servings: 4

Ingredients:

- ½ cup chickpea croutons
- 10 ounces tofu, firmed, drain, dice
- 1 romaine lettuce, chopped
- 1 cup vegan Caesar dressing
- ¼ cup grated vegan
- Parmesan cheese

For the Dressing:

- ½ teaspoon garlic powder
- ½ teaspoon ground black pepper
- ½ teaspoon sweet paprika
- ½ teaspoon onion powder
- ½ teaspoon cumin
- ½ teaspoon dried thyme
- 3 tablespoons soy sauce
- 3 tablespoons water

Directions:

1. Place tofu pieces on a baking sheet lined with baking paper and then bake for 30 minutes at 390 degrees F until golden brown on all sides, turning halfway.
2. Meanwhile, prepare the dressing and for this, place all of its ingredients in a bowl and whisk until smooth.
3. When tofu has roasted, let it cool for 5 minutes, then add to the bowl along with remaining ingredients for the salad, drizzle with prepared dressing and toss until combined.
4. Serve straight away.

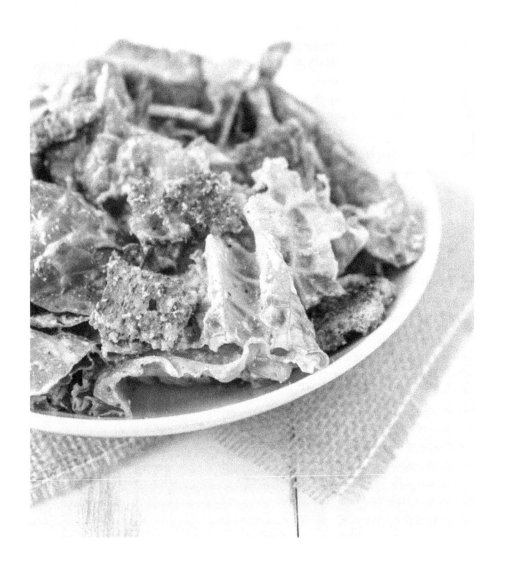

Vegan Chinese Salad

Preparation time: 10 minutes

Cooking time: 0 minute

Servings: 4

Ingredients:

For the Salad:

- 1 iceberg lettuce, chopped
- 1/4 cup soybean sprouts
- 2 carrots, peeled, julienned
- 1/4 cup agar, hydrated

For the Dressing:

- 1/4 teaspoon salt
- 1/4 cup coconut sugar
- 1 tablespoon olive oil
- 1/4 cup apple cider vinegar

Directions:

1. Soak agar in water until hydrated, then drain it and place it in a bowl along with remaining ingredients for the salad.

2. Meanwhile, prepare the dressing and for this, place all of its ingredients in a food processor and pulse until smooth.

3. Drizzle the dressing over the salad, stir until well mixed and then serve.

Heirloom Tomato Salad

Preparation time: 10 minutes

Cooking time: 0 minute

Servings: 6

Ingredients:

For the Salad:

- 1 pound heirloom tomatoes, cut into wedges
- ½ teaspoon salt
- ½ teaspoon ground black pepper
- ¼ cup basil leaves, for serving

For the Dressing:

- 2 cups grape tomatoes, halved
- ¼ teaspoon ground black pepper
- ½ teaspoon salt
- 2 tablespoons chopped chives
- 1 teaspoon honey
- 1/4 cup olive oil
- 2 tablespoons apple cider vinegar

Directions:

1. Prepare the dressing for this, whisk together honey, vinegar, oil, salt, and black pepper until combined, then add chives and tomatoes and toss until combined.

2. Prepare the salad and for this, place tomatoes on a plate, season with salt and black pepper, drizzle with the dressing and top with basil.

3. Serve straight away.

Zucchini Salad

Preparation time: 10 minutes

Cooking time: 15 minutes

Servings: 4

Ingredients:

- 2 cups cubed zucchini
- 1 tablespoon chopped mint
- 1 small white onion, peeled, sliced
- ½ of a lemon, juiced
- 1 teaspoon minced garlic
- 2 tablespoons olive oil
- 1/8 teaspoon ground white pepper
- ¼ teaspoon salt
- 1/8 teaspoon ground turmeric
- 1/2 teaspoon ground cumin
- 7 saffron threads

Directions:

1. Take a skillet pan, place it over medium heat, add oil and when hot, add onion and garlic, and cook for 4 minutes until softened.
2. Then add remaining ingredients, except for salt, black pepper, lime juice, and mint, stir until mixed and cook for 8 minutes until zucchini is tender-crisp.
3. When done, let the salad cool for 10 minutes, then season with salt and black pepper, drizzle with lemon juice, sprinkle with mint and serve

Beet, Mushroom and Avocado Salad

Preparation time: 15 minutes

Cooking time: 20 minutes

Servings: 4

Ingredients:

- 8 ounces cooked beets, chopped
- 4 medium portobello mushroom caps
- 5 ounces baby kale
- 2 medium avocados, pitted, sliced
- 1 small shallot, peeled, chopped
- ¾ teaspoon salt
- ¼ teaspoon ground black pepper
- 1/4 cup lemon juice
- 3 tablespoons olive oil
- 2 sheets of matzo, cut into bite-size pieces

Directions:

1. Place mushroom caps on a baking sheet, spray them with oil, then season them with ½ teaspoon salt and bake for 20 minutes at 450 degrees F until tender.
2. Place shallots in a small bowl, add black pepper and remaining salt, pour in oil and lemon juice and whisk until combined.
3. Place kale and beets in a dish, drizzle with shallot mixture and toss until combined.
4. When mushrooms have roasted, let them cool for 10 minutes, then slice them and to the kale mixture along with remaining ingredients.
5. Toss until well combined and serve.

Tomato Basil Salad

Preparation time: 10 minutes

Cooking time: 0 minute

Servings: 4

Ingredients:

- 3 tablespoons chopped red onion
- 1 pound tomatoes, chopped
- 10 leaves of basil, cut into ribbons
- 1/4 teaspoon ground black pepper
- 1/2 teaspoon salt
- 2 tablespoons white balsamic vinegar

Directions:

1. Take a large bowl, place all the ingredients in it, stir until well combined, and then let it sit for 5 minutes.
2. Refrigerate the salad for a minimum of 2 hours and then serve straight away.

Sweet Potato and Cauliflower Salad

Preparation time: 10 minutes

Cooking time: 30 minutes

Servings: 8

Ingredients:

For the Salad:

- 1 1/2 pound small sweet potatoes, peeled, cut into ½-inch wedges
- 2/3 cup pomegranate seeds
- 1 small head of cauliflower, cut into florets
- 8 cups mixed lettuces
- 1/2 teaspoon salt
- 1/4 teaspoon ground black pepper
- 3 tablespoons olive oil, divided

For the Dressing:

- 4 tablespoons olive oil, divided
- 1/2 teaspoon salt
- 1/4 teaspoon ground black pepper

- 3 tablespoons apple cider vinegar

Directions:

1. Take a baking sheet, place all the vegetables for the salad on it, drizzle with oil, season with salt and black pepper, toss until well coated, and then bake for 30 minutes at 425 degrees F until roasted.
2. Meanwhile, prepare the dressing and for this, place all of its ingredients in a bowl and whisk until combined.
3. When vegetables have roasted, let them cool for 10 minutes, then place them in a large bowl along with remaining ingredients for the salad, drizzle with the dressing and toss until coated.
4. Serve straight away.

Fennel and Asparagus Salad

Preparation time: 10 minutes

Cooking time: 8 minutes

Servings: 4

Ingredients:

For the Salad:

- 1 cup sliced asparagus, trimmed
- 1 large leek, white part sliced in circles only
- 1 medium avocado, pitted, sliced
- 2 cups thinly sliced fennel bulb, trimmed
- 3 tablespoons olive oil
- ¼ cup almonds, toasted

For the Dressing:

- 1 tablespoon thyme
- 2 tablespoons lemon juice
- ¾ teaspoon sea salt
- ½ teaspoon ground black pepper
- 1 teaspoon ground coriander
- 3 tablespoons olive oil

Directions:

1. Prepare the dressing and for this, place all of its ingredients in a bowl and whisk until combined.
2. Sauté leeks in oil for 6 minutes or until it wilts and turns golden brown, then season with some salt and let it cool.
3. Take a large bowl, place all the ingredients for the salad in it, except for almonds, drizzle with the salad dressing and toss until well coated.
4. Top the salad with the almonds and then serve.

Thai Noodle Salad

Preparation time: 10 minutes

Cooking time: 0 minute

Servings: 6

Ingredients:

For the Thai Peanut Sauce:

- 3 thin slices of ginger
- ½ teaspoon salt
- 3 tablespoon lime juice
- 1 clove of garlic, peeled
- 1 teaspoon cayenne pepper
- 2 tablespoons soy sauce
- ¼ cup peanut butter
- 3 tablespoons sesame oil
- ¼ cup of orange juice
- 3 tablespoons honey

For the Salad:

- 6 ounces brown rice noodles, cooked
- 4 cups mix of shredded cabbage, radish, and carrots

- 3 scallions, sliced
- 1 medium red bell pepper, peeled, sliced
- 1 tablespoon jalapeño, chopped
- ½ bunch of cilantro, chopped
- ½ cup roasted peanuts, crushed

Directions:

1. Prepare the sauce, and for this, place all of its ingredients in a blender and pulse until smooth.
2. Take a large bowl, place all the ingredients for the salad in it, except for almonds, top with prepared sauce and toss until well coated.
3. Top the salad with almonds and then serve straight away.

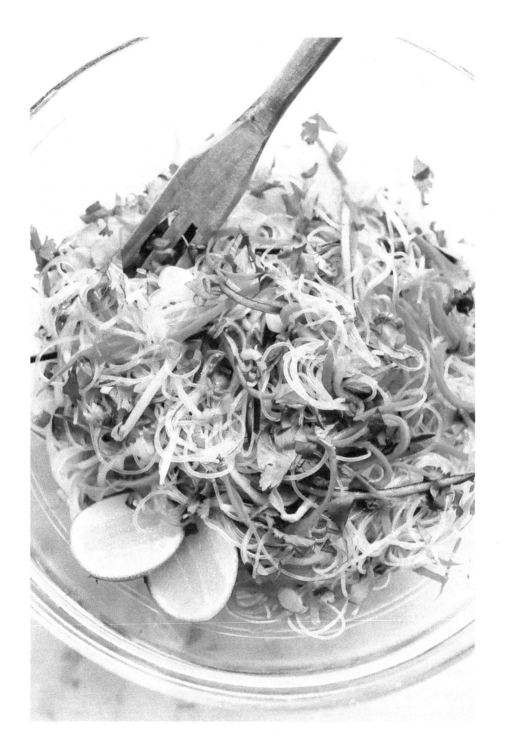

Cherry Tomato and Tofu Salad

Preparation time: 10 minutes

Cooking time: 0 minute

Servings: 2

Ingredients:

For the Salad:

- 2 slices of tofu
- 1 cup cherry tomatoes, halved
- 1 teaspoon sesame seeds

For the Dressing:

- 2 teaspoons soy sauce
- ¼ teaspoon ground black pepper
- ¼ teaspoon of sea salt
- 1 teaspoon sherry vinegar
- 1 teaspoon toasted sesame oil
- 2 tablespoons olive oil

Directions:

1. Prepare the dressing and for this, place all of its ingredients in a small bowl and whisk until smooth.
2. Place cherry tomatoes in a bowl, drizzle with dressing, toss until well coated and sprinkle with sesame seeds.
3. Prepare the salad and for this, place tofu slices on a plate, top with tomato mixture and serve straight away.

Cabbage and Mango Slaw

Preparation time: 20 minutes

Cooking time: 0 minute

Servings: 4

Ingredients:

- 1 jalapeno, chopped
- 3 cups shredded cabbage
- ¼ cup sliced red onion
- 1 large mango, destoned, cubed
- ½ cup chopped cilantro
- ½ teaspoon salt
- 1 orange, juiced, zested
- 2 teaspoons olive oil
- 1 lime, juiced, zested

Directions:

1. Take a large bowl, place all the ingredients in it, and toss until well coated.
2. Let the salad refrigerate for 15 minutes and then serve.

Lentil Tabouli Salad

Preparation time: 5 minutes

Cooking time: 15 minutes

Servings: 4

Ingredients:

For the Salad:

- 1 1/2 cups puy lentils, cooked
- 1/3 cup diced red onion
- 2 cups diced tomatoes
- 1/4 cup chopped mint
- 1 1/2 cups chopped parsley

For the Dressing:

- 1/3 teaspoon ground black pepper
- 1 teaspoon cinnamon
- 1 teaspoon salt
- 2 teaspoon allspice
- 3 tablespoons olive oil
- 1 lemon, juiced, zested

Directions:

1. Prepare the dressing and for this, place all of its ingredients in a small bowl and whisk until smooth.
2. Take a large bowl, place all the ingredients for the salad in it, top with prepared dressing and toss until well coated.
3. Let the salad stand for 10 minutes and then serve

Moroccan Salad with Blood Oranges

Preparation time: 15 minutes

Cooking time: 0 minute

Servings: 4

Ingredients:

- 1 cup quinoa, cooked
- 3 blood oranges, divided
- 2 green onions, sliced
- ¼ cup sliced kalamata olives
- ¼ teaspoon salt
- ¼ teaspoon ground black pepper
- 1 tablespoon apple cider vinegar
- ¼ cup olive oil
- 1 teaspoon honey
- ¼ cup slivered almonds, toasted
- 12 mint leaves, torn

Directions:

1. Take a large bowl, place all the ingredients in it, except the last two ones, and toss until well coated.
2. Top the salad with almonds and mint and then serve straight away.

Cucumber Salad with Chili and Lime

Preparation time: 5 minutes

Cooking time: 0 minute

Servings: 4

Ingredients:

- 1 jalapeno, deseeded, diced
- 2 large cucumbers, sliced
- ¼ of a medium red onion, sliced
- ½ bunch of cilantro
- ½ teaspoon red chili flakes
- 1/2 teaspoon salt
- ½ teaspoon coriander
- 3 tablespoons lime juice
- 2 tablespoons olive oil

Directions:

1. Take a large bowl, place all the ingredients in it, and toss until well coated.

2. Serve straight away

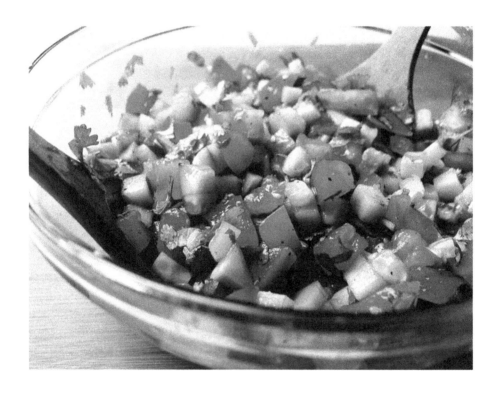

Lemon & Strawberry Soup

Preparation Time:4 hours and 10 minutes

Cooking Time:0 minute

Servings: 4

Ingredients:

- 1 cup buttermilk
- 3 cups strawberries, sliced
- 1 tsp. lemon thyme
- 2 tsp. lemon zest
- 2 tbsp. honey

Directions:

1. Blend the buttermilk and strawberries in your food processor.
2. Transfer this mixture to a bowl.
3. Add the thyme and lemon zest.
4. Chill in the refrigerator for 4 hours.
5. Strain the soup and stir in the honey.
6. Serve in bowls.

Bursting Black Bean Soup

Servings: 6

Preparation time: 8 hours and 10 minutes

Ingredients:

- 1 pound of black beans, uncooked
- 1/4 cup of lentils, uncooked
- 1 medium-sized carrot, peeled and chopped
- 2 medium-sized green bell peppers, cored and chopped
- 1 stalk of celery, chopped
- 28 ounce of diced tomatoes
- 2 jalapeno pepper, seeded and minced
- 1 large red onion, peeled and chopped
- 3 teaspoons of minced garlic
- 1 tablespoon of salt
- 1/2 teaspoon ground black pepper
- 2 tablespoons of red chili powder
- 2 teaspoons of ground cumin
- 1/2 teaspoon of dried oregano
- 3 tablespoons of apple cider vinegar
- 1/2 cup of brown rice, uncooked
- 3 quarts of water, divided

Directions:

1. Place a large pot over medium-high heat, add the beans, pour in 1 1/2 quarts of water and boil it.
2. Let it boil for 10 minutes, then remove the pot from the heat, let it stand for 1 hour and then cover the pot.
3. Drain the beans and add it to a 6-quarts slow cooker.
4. Pour in the remaining 1 1/2 quarts of water and cover it with the lid.
5. Plug in the slow cooker and let it cook for 3 hours at the high setting or until it gets soft.
6. When the beans are done, add the remaining ingredients except for the rice and continue cooking for 3 hours on the low heat setting.
7. When it is30 minutes left to finish, add the rice to the slow cooker and let it cook.
8. When done, using an immersion blender process half of the soup and then serve.

Portobello Onion Burgers

Preparation time: 10 minutes

Cooking time: 30 minutes

Servings 2 burgers

Ingredients:

- 1 large green onion, cut into rings
- 2 tablespoons olive oil
- 2 Portobello mushrooms
- 1 teaspoon balsamic vinegar
- 1/8 teaspoon chili flakes
- 1 teaspoon agave syrup
- 1 teaspoon soy sauce
- Salt, pepper (to taste)

Directions:

1. Add one tablespoon of olive oil to frying pan and heat over low. Sauté onions for approximately 20 minutes, until tender.
2. After cooked, add chili flakes.

3. In a large mixing bowl, create a sauce by combining soy sauce, balsamic vinegar, agave syrup, and salt/pepper.
4. Coat the mushrooms evenly with this sauce.
5. Add one tablespoon of olive oil to frying pan and heat over medium.
6. Cook burgers on each side 7 minutes, until golden brown.

Tofu Almond Burgers

Preparation time: 10 minutes

Cooking time: 30 minutes

Servings 6–8 burgers

Ingredients:

- 2 tablespoons flax seeds, freshly ground
- 4 tablespoons water
- 1 package firm tofu, crumbled
- 1 carrot, peeled and grated
- 2 green onions, finely chopped
- 2 tablespoons sesame oil
- 1 teaspoon grated ginger
- 2 garlic cloves, minced
- 2/3 cup slivered almonds, toasted
- 2 teaspoons soy sauce
- 1 tablespoon sesame seeds

Directions:

1. In a small mixing bowl, combine flax seed and water.

2. Pour sesame oil in a large skillet and warm on low heat.

3. Sauté green onion, carrot, garlic and ginger for 4–5 minutes, until tender.

4. In a large mixing bowl, add remaining ingredient list, flax seed mixture, sautéed items and combine.

5. Using wet hands, form the mixture into a burger shape.

6. Add one tablespoon of olive oil to frying pan and heat over medium.

7. Cook burgers on each side 6 minutes, until golden brown.

Mushroom Chickpea Burgers

Preparation time: 10 minutes

Cooking time: 50 minutes

Servings 6–8 burgers

Ingredients:

- 2 cups mushrooms, finely chopped
- 1 onion, chopped
- 2 garlic cloves, minced
- 1 teaspoon curry powder
- 1 cup canned chickpeas, drained
- 2 carrots, peeled and grated
- 2 tablespoons chopped coriander
- 2 tablespoons flour
- Salt, pepper (to taste)

Directions:

1. In a medium size frying pan, heat one tablespoon of olive oil and sauté onion and garlic for approximately 2 minutes.

2. Add curry, carrots and mushrooms, turn heat down to low and continue to cook for ten minutes.
3. Set aside.
4. In a food processor, pulse the chickpeas until a paste forms.
5. In a large mixing bowl, combine the mushroom mixture an the paste.
6. Stir in coriander, flour, and salt/pepper.
7. Wet your hands and mold mixture into a burger shape.
8. Add one tablespoon of olive oil to a frying pan on medium heat.
9. Burger will be cooked thoroughly when both sides are a golden brown.
10. Serve on your favorite bread, using toppings of your choice and tastiest condiments.

Summer Chickpea Salad

Serves: 4

Preparation Time: 15 Minutes

Ingredients:

- 1 ½ Cups Cherry Tomatoes, Halved
- 1 Cup English Cucumber, Slices
- 1 Cup Chickpeas, Canned, Unsalted, Drained & Rinsed
- ¼ Cup Red Onion, Slivered
- 2 Tablespoon Olive Oil
- 1 ½ Tablespoons Lemon Juice, Fresh
- 1 ½ Tablespoons Lemon Juice, Fresh
- Sea Salt & Black Pepper to Taste

Directions:

1. Mix everything together, and toss to combine before serving.

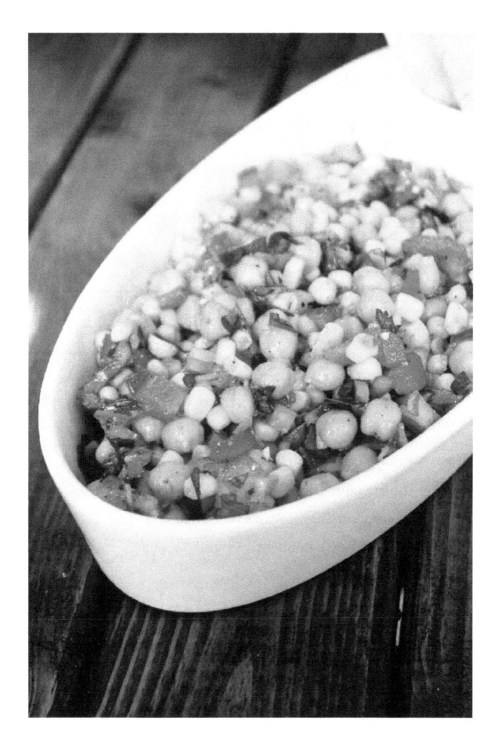

Fruity Kale Salad

Serves: 4

Preparation Time: 30 Minutes

Ingredients:

Salad:

- 10 Ounces Baby Kale
- ½ Cup Pomegranate Arils
- 1 Tablespoon Olive
- Oil 1 Apple, Sliced

Dressing:

- 3 Tablespoons Apple Cider Vinegar
- 3 Tablespoons Olive Oil
- 1 Tablespoon Tahini Sauce (Optional)
- Sea Salt & Black Pepper to Taste

Directions:

2. Wash and dry the kale.
3. If kale is too expensive, you can also use lettuce, arugula or spinach.

4. Take the stems out, and chop it.
5. Combine all of your salad ingredients together.
6. Combine all of your dressing ingredients together before drizzling it over the salad to serve.

Avocado & Radish Salad

Serves: 2

Preparation Time: 10 Minutes

Ingredients:

- 1 Avocado, Sliced
- 6 Radishes, Sliced
- 2 Tomatoes, Sliced
- 1 Lettuce Head, Leaves Separated
- ½ Red Onion, Peeled & Sliced

Dressing:

- ½ Cup Olive Oil
- ¼ Cup Lime Juice, Fresh
- ¼ Cup Apple Cider Vinegar
- 3 Cloves Garlic, Chopped
- Fine Sea Salt & Black Pepper to Taste

Directions:

1. Spread your lettuce leaves on a platter, and then layer with your onion, tomatoes, avocado and radishes.

2. Whisk your dressing ingredients together before drizzling it over your salad.

Interesting Facts:

Avocados themselves are ranked within the top five of the healthiest foods on the planet, so you know that the oil that is produced from them is too. It is loaded with healthy fats and essential fatty acids. Like race bran oil it is perfect to cook with as well! Bonus: Helps in the prevention of diabetes and lowers cholesterol levels.

Watercress & Blood Orange

Salad Serves: 4

Preparation Time: 10 Minutes

Ingredients:

- 1 Tablespoon Hazelnuts, Toasted & Chopped
- 2 Blood Oranges (or Navel Oranges)
- 3 Cups watercress, Stems Removed
- 1/8 Teaspoon Sea Salt, Fine
- 1 Tablespoon Lemon Juice, Fresh
- 1 Tablespoon Honey, Raw
- 1 Tablespoon Water
- 2 Tablespoons Chives, Fresh

Directions:

1. Whisk your oil, honey, lemon juice, chives, salt and water together.
2. Add in your watercress, tossing until it's coated.
3. Arrange the mixture onto salad plates, and top with orange slices.

4. Drizzle with remaining liquid, and sprinkle with hazelnuts.

Interesting Facts:

Lemons are popularly known as harboring loads of Vitamin C, but are also excellent sources of folate, fiber, and antioxidants. Bonus: Helps lower cholesterol. Double Bonus: Reduces risk of cancer and high blood pressure.

Tzatziki

Preparation Time: 20minutes

Ingredients:

- 1 cup of natural vegan yogurt
- 1/4 cucumber (grated)
- 1 tablespoon of fresh dill
- 1 teaspoon of lemon peel
- 1 tablespoon of Nutritional yeast
- 1 tsp black pepper
- 1 teaspoon of salt
- 1 chopped clove of garlic
- 1 tablespoon of olive oil
- 1 tablespoon of lemon juice

Directions:

1. Preparation Mix all INGREDIENTS in a medium bowl.

2. Stir together.

3. Place on a serving plate, cover well and refrigerate up to 1 hour before serving.

Fish sauce

Preparation Time: 30minutes

Ingredients:

- 1/2 cup grated wakame (see notes)
- 2 cups of filtered water
- 2 large cloves of garlic, crushed
- 1 teaspoon of whole peppercorns
- 1/3 cup of dark soy sauce with mushroom flavor, normal soy sauce or gluten-free tamari
- 1 teaspoon of Genmai Miso (it's quite salty, so optional)

Directions:

1. Combine the wakame, garlic, peppercorns and water in a large pan and cook.
2. Lower the heat and simmer for about twenty minutes.
3. Strain and return the liquid to the pot.
4. Add the soy sauce, cook again and cook until the mixture is almost salty and unbearable.
5. Remove from the heat and add miso.
6. Transfer to a bottle and keep in the fridge.
7. Use one by one to replace fish sauce in vegan recipes.

Creamy cucumber herb

Preparation Time: 10minutes

Ingredients:

- 3 ounces of cashew nuts, soaked in water for 2 hours
- 2 1/2 ounces of cucumber, peeled and chopped
- 1/4 cup of unsweetened milk
- 1/2 ounce chopped shallot
- 1/2 lemon juice
- 1 small clove of garlic, peeled
- 1 teaspoon of apple cider vinegar
- 1/2 teaspoon of salt
- 1/4 tsp garlic powder
- A pinch of ground black pepper
- 1 tablespoon of finely chopped fresh dill
- 1 tablespoon of finely chopped fresh parsley
- 1 tablespoon of finely chopped fresh chives

Directions:

1. Add all the INGREDIENTS except herbs in a small blender and mix to a creamy and smooth consistency.

2. Add the herbs and mix well.

Roasted Vegetables in Balsamic Sauce

Preparation Time: 10 minutes

Cooking Time: 23 minutes

Servings: 12

Ingredients:

- 1 onion, sliced into wedges
- 2 cloves garlic, minced
- 1 lb. green beans, trimmed
- 2 tablespoons olive oil
- Salt and pepper to taste
- 4 yellow summer squash, sliced
- ⅔ cup balsamic vinegar

Directions:

1. Preheat your oven to 450 degrees F.
2. Toss onion, garlic and beans in olive oil.
3. Transfer to a baking pan.
4. Season with salt and pepper.

5. Roast in the oven for 8 minutes.

6. Add the squash.

7. Roast for another 5 minutes.

8. Transfer roasted vegetables in a food container.

9. Reheat the veggies and toss in balsamic vinegar sauce when ready to serve.

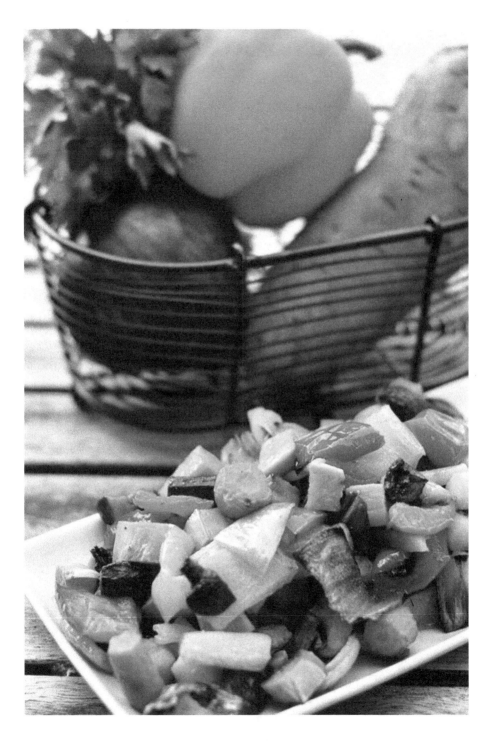

Vegetable Salad in Mason Sauce

Preparation Time: 5 minutes

Cooking Time: 0 minute

Servings: 1

Ingredients:

- 2 tablespoons cashew sauce (recipe in the sauce section)

- 1 cup tofu cubes, roasted

- 1 tablespoon pumpkin seeds

- 1 cup carrots, roasted

- 2 cups mixed greens

Directions:

1. In a glass jar, layer the cashew sauce, tofu, seeds, carrots and mixed greens.

2. Seal the jar.

3. Refrigerate up to 5 days.

4. Serve whenever ready to eat.

Mixed herbs with almonds and pepita pesto

Preparation Time: 30minutes

Ingredients:

- 1 cup wrapped fresh basil leaves
- 1 cup wrapped arugula
- 2 cloves garlic (grated)
- 1/2 cup raw pepita
- 1/4 cup raw almonds
- 1/4 cup fresh lemon juice
- 2 tbsp virgin olive oil
- 1/2 tsp salt (or to taste)
- 1/8 teaspoon pepper (or to taste)
- 2-3 tbsp of thin water

Directions:

1. Place all INGREDIENTS except olive oil and water in a food processor.
2. Processing Before combining, split sides as needed.

3. Sprinkle olive oil on top while the machine is still running.
4. This should work smoothly.
5. Add Water 1 Ch.
6. Simultaneously process after each addition and scroll through the pages as needed until you reach the desired consistency.

Diluted banana caramel sauce

Preparation Time: 30minutes

Ingredients:

- 2 large very ripe bananas
- 1/4 cup coconut sugar (use 1/2 cup if your banana is not too ripe or you like sweet sides)
- 2 tbsp brown rice syrup
- 1/2 cup milk milk
- 1 teaspoon pure vanilla extract
- 1/4 tsp salt

Directions:

1. Put all INGREDIENTS in a blender or food processor and puree for a few seconds until smooth.
2. Pour the mixture into the baking sheet and bring to a boil.

3. You may need to adjust the heat as it burns.

4. You don't want to burn sugar, but you want a good bladder to reduce it.

5. The mixture will be ready when it is reduced by about half.

Zucchini Soup

Preparation Time: 5 minutes

Cooking Time: 15 minutes

Servings: 4

Ingredients:

- 3 cups chicken broth
- 1 tbsp. tarragon, chopped
- 3 zucchinis, sliced
- 3 oz. cheddar cheese
- Salt and pepper to taste

Directions:

1. Pour the broth into a pot. Stir in the tarragon and zucchini.
2. Bring to a boil and then simmer for 10 minutes.
3. Transfer to a blender and blend until smooth.
4. Put it back to the stove and stir in cheese.
5. Season with salt and pepper.

Corn & Black Bean Salad

Salad: 6

Time: 10 Minutes

Ingredients:

- ¼ Cup Cilantro, Fresh & Chopped
- 1 Can Corn, Drained (10 Ounces)
- 1/8 Cup Red Onion, Chopped
- 1 Can Black Beans, Drained (15 Ounces)
- 1 Tomato, Chopped
- 3 Tablespoons Lemon Juice, Fresh
- 2 Tablespoons Olive Oil
- Sea Salt & Black Pepper to Taste

Directions:

1. Mix everything together, and then refrigerate until cool.
2. Serve cold.

Interesting Facts: Whole corn is a fantastic source of phosphorus, magnesium, and B vitamins. It also promotes healthy digestion and contains heart-healthy antioxidants. It is important to seek out organic corn in order to bypass all of the genetically modified product that is out on the market.

Red Pepper & Broccoli Salad

Serves: 2

Time: 15 Minutes

Calories: 185 | Protein: 4 Grams | Fat: 14 Grams | Carbs: 8 Grams

Ingredients:

- Ounces Lettuce Salad Mix
- 1 Head Broccoli, Chopped into Florets
- 1 Red Pepper, Seeded & Chopped

Dressing:

- 3 Tablespoons White Wine Vinegar
- 1 Teaspoon Dijon Mustard
- 1 Clove Garlic, Peeled & Chopped Fine
- ½ Teaspoon Black Pepper
- ½ Teaspoon Sea Salt, Fine
- 2 Tablespoons Olive Oil
- 1 Tablespoon Parsley, Chopped

Directions:

1. In boiling water, drain the broccoli it on a paper towel.
2. Whisk together all dressing ingredients.
3. Toss ingredients together before serving.

Interesting Facts:

This oil is the main source of dietary fat in a variety of diets. It contains many vitamins and minerals that play a part in reducing the risk of stroke and lowers cholesterol and high blood pressure and can also aid in weight loss. It is best consumed cold, as when it is heated it can lose some of its nutritive properties (although it is still great to cook with – extra virgin is best), many recommend taking a shot of cold oil olive daily! Bonus: if you don't like the taste or texture add a shot to your smoothie.

Cheesy Asparagus Pasta

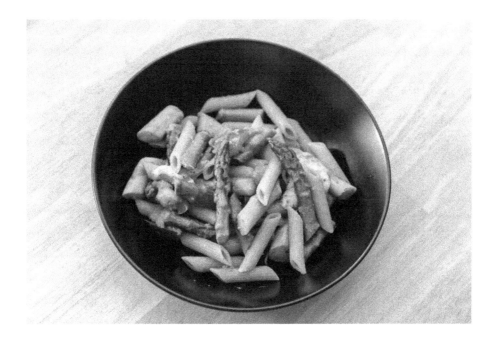

Preparation time: 10 minutes

Cooking time: 50 minutes

Servings: 4

Ingredients:

- 2 Cups Pasta
- 1 Cup Vegan Cheese, Shredded
- 3 ½ Cups Vegetable Broth

- ½ Cup Vegan Alfredo Sauce
- 6 Asparagus Spears, Chopped

Directions:

1. Mix your pasta, broth and asparagus in your instant pot.
2. Seal the lid, and cook on high pressure for seven minutes.
3. Use a quick release, and rain your pasta.
4. Add it all back into the cooker, and then stir in the sauce and cheese.
5. Sauté for two minutes before serving warm.

Kale & Mushroom

Preparation time: 10 minutes

Cooking time: 40 minutes

Servings: 4

Ingredients:

- 1 Tablespoon Olive Oil
- 1 Sweet Onion, Diced
- 2 Cloves Garlic, Minced
- 1 lb. Baby Bella Mushrooms, Sliced
- 1 Tomato, Diced
- 1 Teaspoon Smoked Paprika
- Sea Salt & Black Pepper to Taste
- 1 Bay Leaf
- 3 Cups Campanella Pasta
- 3 ¼ Cups Vegetable Stock
- 1 Cup Cashew Sour Cream
- 3 Cups Kale, Rinsed & Torn

Directions:

1. Press sauté and then add the oil.
2. Once it's hot cook the onion for two minutes, while stirring frequently.
3. Add the garlic, cooking for another minute and stir well.
4. Add the tomato, paprika, bay leaf, mushrooms and salt.
5. Allow it to sit for three minutes.
6. Stir in the pasta and stock, and then lock your lid.
7. Cook on high pressure for three minutes.
8. Allow for a natural pressure release for five minutes and then finish with a quick release.
9. Discard the bay leaf, and sauté for two more minutes if there is excess liquid.
10. Stir in the kale and sour cream, allowing your kale to wilt for two minutes.
11. Season with salt before serving.

Edamame & Aleppo Pepper

Preparation Time: 5 minutes

Cooking Time: 5 minutes

Serving: 1

Ingredients:

- ½ cup edamame pods
- Water ⅛ teaspoon
- Aleppo pepper

Directions:

1. Place edamame pods in a steamer basket.
2. Put the basket on top of a pot with water.
3. Steam.
4. Store in glass jar with lid.
5. Season with Aleppo pepper before serving.

Clarissa

Preparation Time: 30minutes

Ingredients:

- 1/4 cup of dried red cayenne pepper
- 20 soft red peppers like Byadgi or Wide Chili (also dried)
- 1 1/2 tablespoons of cumin
- 1 teaspoon of coriander seeds
- 4 cloves of garlic
- 1 teaspoon of salt
- 3 tablespoons of olive oil
- 1/4 cup fresh coriander
- 1 tablespoon of chopped mint (optional)

Directions:

1. Soak the chillies with 1/2 cup of warm water for 15 minutes.
2. Drain and keep water.
3. Meanwhile, roasted cumin and coriander.
4. Grind the powder in a coffee grinder.

5. Put the paprika, ground spices, garlic, salt and olive oil in a blender with a little water and cut into a paste.

6. Add the chopped coriander and mint and press several times.

7. Use a little more water if necessary.

8. Store the mixture in the refrigerator then use as needed.

Toasted Banana Caramel Sauce

Preparation Time: 30minutes

Ingredients:

- 2 large ripe bananas
- 1/4 cup coconut sugar (use 1/2 cup if your bananas are not overripe or if you like sweeter things)
- 2 tbsp brown rice syrup
- 1/2 cup milk without milk
- 1 tsp pure vanilla extract
- 1/4 teaspoon salt

Directions:

1. Put all INGREDIENTS in a blender or food processor and beat for a few seconds until smooth.
2. Pour the mixture into a pan and bring to a boil.

3. Reduce heat and simmer for 20 minutes, stirring constantly.

4. It may be necessary to adjust the heat as it boils.

5. You don't want sugars to burn, but you want a good bubble to occur so that it shrinks.

6. The mixture is ready when it is halved.

Mushroom Pineapple Burgers

Preparation time: 10 minutes

Cooking time: 40 minutes

Servings 2 burgers

Ingredients:

- 2 Portobello mushrooms
- 2 slices fresh pineapple
- 1/4 cup teriyaki sauce
- 1 teaspoon agave syrup
- Salt, pepper
- Vegan burger buns

Directions:

- Create a sauce by combining teriyaki sauce, agave syrup, and salt/pepper.
- Brush the sauce over mushrooms and pineapple, coating evenly.
- Add one tablespoon of olive oil to frying pan and heat over medium.

- Cook mushrooms on each side 7 minutes, until golden brown.
- Heat pineapple in pan with mushrooms until cooked through.
- Using the vegan burger bun for serving, layer mushrooms and pineapple and enjoy!

Parsley Salad

Serves: 8

Preparation Time: 30 Minutes

Ingredients:

- 3 Lemons, Juiced
- 150 Grams Flat Lea Parsley, Chopped Fine
- 1 Cup Boiled Water
- 5 Tablespoons Olive Oil
- Sea Salt & Black Pepper to Taste
- 6 Green Onions, Chopped Fine
- 1 Cup Bulgur
- 4 Tomatoes, Chopped Fine

Directions:

1. Add your Bulgur to your water, and mix well.
2. Put a towel on top of it to steam it.
3. Keep it to the side, and then chop your spring onions, tomatoes and parsley.
4. Put them in your salad bowl.

5. Pour your juice into the mixture, and then add in your olive oil, salt and pepper.

6. Put this mixture over your bulgur to serve.

Chunky Black Lentil Veggie Soup

Servings: 8

Preparation time: 4 hours and 35 minutes

Ingredients:

- 1 1/2 cups of black lentils, uncooked
- 2 small turnips, peeled and diced
- 10 medium-sized carrots, peeled and diced
- 1 medium-sized green bell pepper, cored and diced
- 3 cups of diced tomatoes
- 1 medium-sized white onion, peeled and diced
- 2 tablespoons of minced ginger
- 1 teaspoon of minced garlic
- 1 teaspoon of salt
- 1/2 teaspoon of ground coriander
- 1/2 teaspoon of ground cumin
- 3 tablespoons of unsalted butter
- 32 fluid ounce of vegetable broth
- 32 fluid ounce of water

Directions:

- Using a medium-sized microwave, cover the bowl, place the lentils and pour in the water.
- Microwave lentils for 10 minutes or until softened, stirring after 5 minutes.
- Drain lentils and add to a 6-quarts slow cooker along with remaining ingredients and stir until just mix.
- Cover with top, plug in slow cooker; adjust cooking time to 6 hours and let cook on low heat setting or until carrots are tender.
- Serve straight away.

Celery Salad

Preparation time: 10 minutes

Serves: 6

Ingredients:

- 6 cups celery, sliced
- ¼ tsp celery seed
- 1 tbsp lemon juice
- 2 tsp lemon zest, grated
- 1 tbsp parsley, chopped
- 1 tbsp olive oil
- Sea salt

Directions:

1. Add all ingredients into the large mixing bowl and toss well.
2. Serve immediately and enjoy.

Red Bell Pepper Salad

Preparation Time: 10 minutes

Cooking Time: 10 minutes

Servings: 4

Ingredients:

- 4 red bell peppers, sliced into quarters
- 4 oz. mozzarella cheese
- 3 tbsp. basil, chopped
- 1 tbsp. balsamic glaze
- 1 ½ tbsp. olive oil
- Salt and pepper to taste

Directions:

1. Preheat your broiler.
2. Broil the bell peppers for 10 minutes.
3. Toss with the mozzarella and basil.
4. Drizzle with the balsamic glaze and olive oil.
5. Season with salt and pepper.

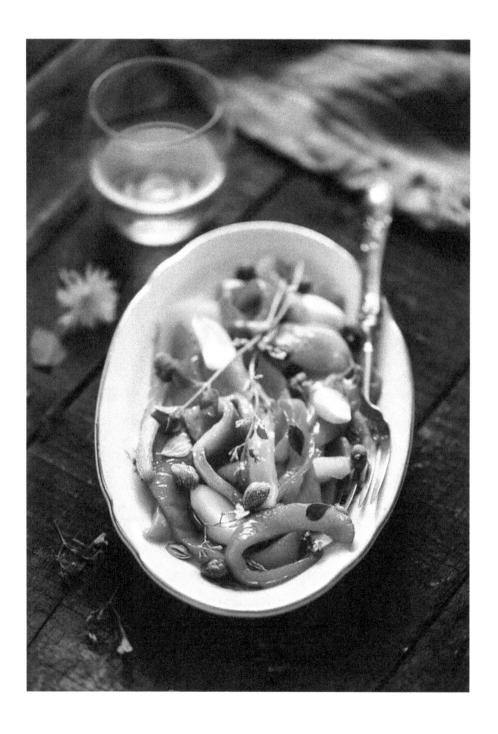

Parsnip & Split Pea Soup

Servings: 8

Preparation time: 5 hours and 10 minutes

Ingredients:

- 1 tablespoon of olive oil
- 2 large parsnips, peeled and chopped
- 2 large carrots, peeled and chopped
- 1 medium-sized white onion, peeled and diced
- 1 1/2 teaspoon of minced garlic
- 2 1/4 cups of dried green split peas, rinsed
- 1 teaspoon of salt
- 1/2 teaspoon of ground black pepper
- 1 teaspoon of dried thyme
- 2 bay leaves
- 6 cups of vegetable broth
- 1 teaspoon of liquid smoke

Directions:

1. Place a medium-sized non-stick skillet pan over an average pressure of heat, add the oil and let it heat.

2. Add the parsnip, carrot, onion, garlic and let it cook for 5 minutes or until it is heated.
3. Transfer this mixture into a 6-quarts slow cooker and add the remaining ingredients.
4. Stir until mixes properly and cover the top.
5. Plug in the slow cooker; adjust the cooking time to 5 hours and let it cook on the high heat setting or until the peas and vegetables get soft.
6. When done, remove the bay leaf from the soup and blend it with a submersion blender or until the soup reaches your desired state.
7. Add the seasoning and serve.

Chopped Cucumber, Tomato & Radish Salad

Preparation Time: 15 minutes

Cooking Time: 0 minute

Servings: 6

Ingredients:

- 1 tbsp. lemon juice
- ½ cup feta cheese, crumbled
- ½ cup mayonnaise
- Salt and pepper to taste
- 1 tbsp. fresh dill, chopped
- 1 tbsp. fresh chives, chopped
- 1 cucumber, diced
- 3 cups cherry tomatoes, chopped
- 2 cups radish, diced
- 1 onion, minced

Directions:

1. Mix the lemon juice, feta cheese, mayo, salt, pepper, dill and chives in a bowl.
2. Stir in the rest of the ingredients.
3. Toss to coat evenly.

Creamy Creamed Corn

Servings: 5

Preparation time: 4 hours

Ingredients:

- 16 ounce of frozen corn kernels

- 1 teaspoon of salt

- 1/2 teaspoon of ground black pepper

- 1 tablespoon honey

- 1/2 cup of vegetarian butter, unsalted

- 8-ounce of cream cheese, softened

- 1/2 cup of almond milk

Directions:

1. Take a 6-quarts slow cooker, grease it with a non-stick cooking spray and place ingredients in it.

2. Stir properly and cover the top.

3. Plug in the slow cooker; adjust the cooking time to 4 hours and let it cook on the low heat setting or until it is cooked thoroughly.

4. Serve right away.

Creamy Garlic Cauliflower Mashed Potatoes

Servings: 6

Preparation time: 3 hours

Ingredients:

- 30-ounce of cauliflower head, cut into florets
- 6 garlic cloves, peeled
- 1 teaspoon of salt
- 3/4 teaspoon of ground black pepper
- 1 bay leaf
- 1 tablespoon of vegetarian butter, unsalted
- 3 cups of water

Directions:

1. Take a 6-quarts slow cooker, grease it with a non-stick cooking spray and place the cauliflower florets into it.
2. Add the remaining ingredients except for the butter and stir properly.

3. Cover the top, plug in the slow cooker; adjust the cooking time to 3 hours and let it cook on the high heat setting or until it is cooked thoroughly.
4. When done, open the slow cooker, remove the bay leaf and garlic cloves.
5. Drain the cooking liquid, add the butter and let it melt.
6. Then using an immersion blender, mash the cauliflower or until it gets creamy.
7. Add the seasoning and serve.

Healthy Cabbage Soup

Servings: 6

Preparation time: 4 hours and 15 minutes

Ingredients:

- 5 cups of shredded cabbage
- 3 medium-sized carrots, peeled and chopped
- 3 1/2 cups of diced tomatoes
- 1 medium-sized white onion, chopped
- 2 teaspoons of minced garlic
- 1 teaspoon of salt
- 1 teaspoon of dried oregano
- 1 tablespoon of dried parsley
- 1 1/2 cups of tomato sauce
- 5 cups of vegetable broth

Directions:

1. Using a 6-quarts slow cooker, place all the ingredients and stir properly.

2. Cover it with the lid, plug in the slow cooker and let it cook for 4 hours at the high heat setting or until the vegetables are tender.
3. Serve right away.

Tricolore Salad

Preparation Time: 10 minutes

Servings: 5

Ingredients:

- 1 avocado, peeled
- ½ cup kalamata olives
- 2 tablespoon olive oil
- 1 teaspoon minced garlic
- ¼ teaspoon salt
- 2 tomatoes, chopped
- 1 teaspoon apple cider vinegar
- 6 oz Provolone cheese, chopped

Directions:

1. Mix up together salt, apple cider vinegar, minced garlic, and olive oil.
2. Cut kalamata olives into halves.
3. Slice avocado and place in salad bowl.
4. Add olive halves, chopped tomato, and cheese.
5. Stir gently and sprinkle with olive oil mixture.

Florentine

Preparation Time: 10 minutes

Cooking time: 15 minutes

Servings: 4

Ingredients:

- 1 teaspoon butter
- 4 eggs
- 8 oz Edam cheese, shredded
- 1 teaspoon ground paprika
- ¼ teaspoon cayenne pepper
- 2 tablespoon cream cheese

Directions:

1. Preheat oven to 360F.
2. Preheat the springform pan in the oven.
3. Then grease it with butter.
4. Beat the eggs in the greased pan and sprinkle with cayenne pepper.
5. Top eggs with shredded cheese and spread with cream cheese.

6. Sprinkle the meal with ground paprika.

7. Put it in the oven and cook for 15 minutes or until cheese is light brown at 355F.

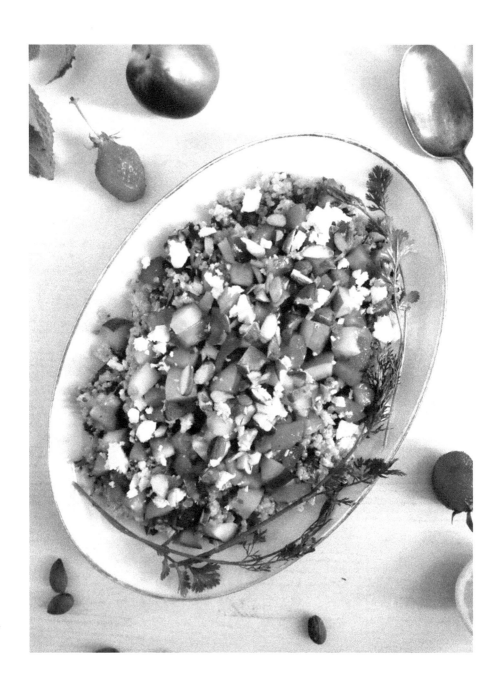

CPSIA information can be obtained
at www.ICGtesting.com
Printed in the USA
BVHW091210130521
607267BV00011B/1469

9 781802 772685